Clean Eating Cookbook for Dummies

Clean Eating 30-day Meal Plan. Easy and Healthy Low Carb Recipes for Weight Loss

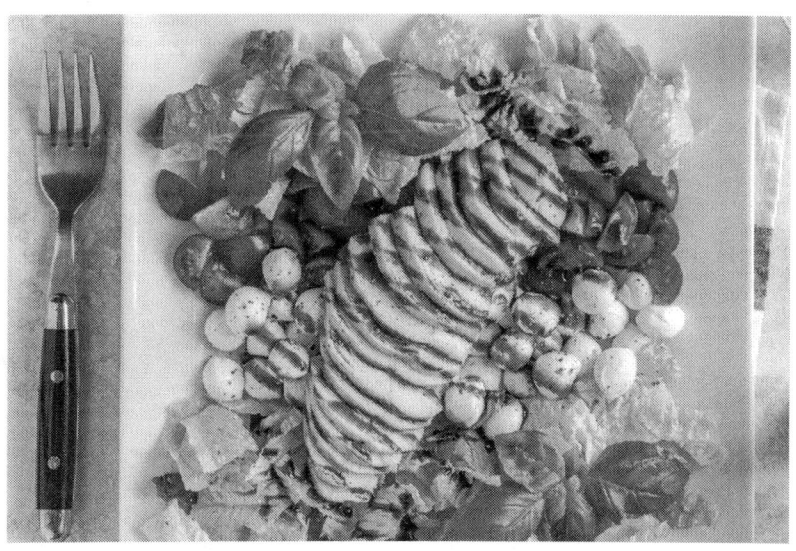

Alice Newman

DEDICATION

I dedicate this book to my all people that want to change their bodies and health and lives

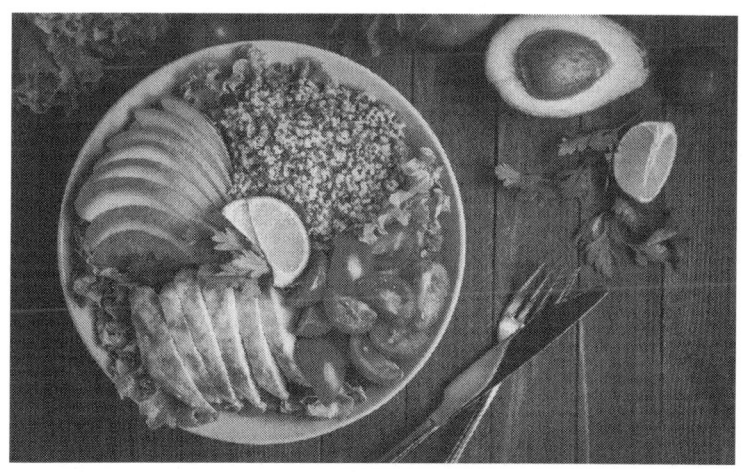

Table of Content

INTRODUCTION

Clean eating has known many definitions through the years, and they all come from how people define the word "clean." Body builders have one definition, your food coach has another, a vegan can surely find a different one, and your doctor will find a new way to define the word as well. Though, the truth is somewhere in between so let's look at the facts and draw our conclusions:

A diet often defines a period that has certain food restrictions with the sole purpose of losing weight or fixing a health problem. A diet is short-term thinking, and it provides a short-term fix. But clean eating is quite the opposite – it has to become a lifestyle for it to work, focusing on a long-term purpose rather than seeing just the short-term benefits.

There are no calorie restrictions. We all know how annoying, frustrating and time-consuming counting calories can be, but clean eating has none of this. Instead, it allows you to eat as much as you want and need to be healthy and have enough energy to do your daily tasks.

There is no food deprivation. How many times have you been on a diet forbidding you to eat a food, ruling out your favorite meat or vegetable, and not even thinking about dessert?! Far too many times! And it's time to change that! Clean eating is not supposed to be a sacrifice or a chore. It's about finding healthy alternatives to unhealthy food. Let's say you love cake – why to give it up?! You can easily find a healthier alternative and enjoy it as much as you would with any other cake.

You can eat as many times a day as you want. No more eating at certain hours or counting the minutes until you can have another tiny snack. Clean eating doesn't focus on that – it's your personal choice how many meals a day you have if they are healthy and packed with nutrients, not just calories to keep you full.

Guidelines are not rules. Unlike diets, clean eating doesn't have strict rules. Instead, it has what I call guidelines – they are there just to guide you and teach you how to live a healthier life, instead of forcing you to comply with rules, which we all never know works!

CHAPTER 1: WHAT IS CLEAN EATING?

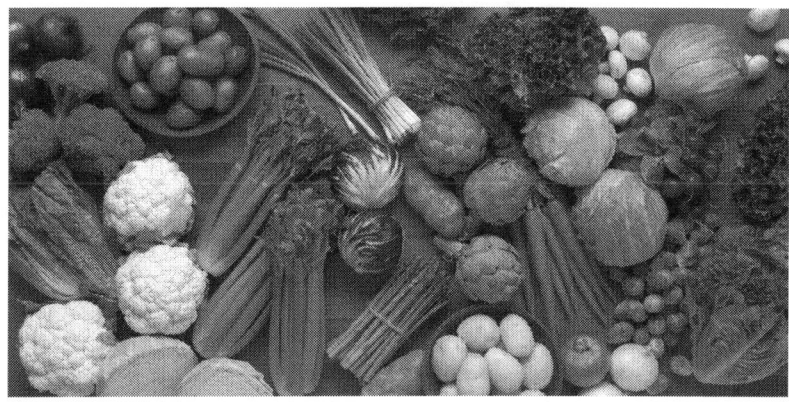

The concept of clean eating revolves around the idea of focusing one's diet on food items that have been through a shorter processing time from the source to your plate. It is about using whole foods to replenish the system real food items that have been minimally handled or refined before making their way to the store shelves.

Being mindful of the ingredients' pathways enables clean eaters to enjoy various products in their most natural and healthiest forms. But with modern innovations revolutionizing the food production process, it can be quite a challenge to eat, let alone source whole foods for daily consumption, with one of the major hurdles being the cost involved. Clean eating means trying to avoid food items that contain artificial components from colorings to flavorings. Substitutes for sugar are also included in the list of things to avoid. The overall goal is for a clean eater to be rid of anything that can compromise one's health.

Many believe that clean eating is difficult, but the rules of the game are rather simple. You can eat anything you wish as long as you are ingesting healthy food. There are no bans on carbs, sugars, or anything that significantly slows down your brain activity, and this makes it an ideal diet for those who want to lose weight or live healthier lives.

Where Did Clean Eating Begin?

Although clean eating focuses on eating food items the way humans have always done, it has been turned into a relatively modern concept of renewing past practices to overcome the excessive lifestyles brought about by evolution and technological advancements.

This excess can be seen in the growing preference for people to have more of everything even if having more is technically unhealthy. The attitude to have more physical belongings is also reflective in the desire to eat more. Obesity, heart disease, stroke, diabetes, and other preventable health issues are becoming prevalent across the world because of this mindset. And this is the kind of attitude that clean eating wants to change.

Is It Just Like Other Unsustainable Diet Fads?

The great thing about clean eating is that it is not a mere diet fad. It is not something people can or should jump into for the sake of quick weight loss. Clean eating calls for a complete change in one's diet. And although short- term goal setting is a part of the process, the primary focus concentrates on the long-term effects of the diet.

Other foods are considered fads because people try them for a couple of days to several weeks and then stop and return to their usual eating habits. These diets are unsustainable because most of them starve people or reduce their mental activity. Clean eating allows you to eat until you are satisfied without compromising your health goals, being more of a lifestyle than a diet.

It also doesn't call for quick and immediate changes to the way you eat. You can start by changing one meal from your daily menu and work from there. The slower and more relaxed integration of new food items makes it easier for people to shift eating habits because the body can adjust to every new change.

The Basic Principles of Clean Eating

It is relatively easy to understand the concept of clean eating. Here are some of its basic principles:

Prioritize Unrefined Foods Over Refined Products.

It will be challenging, but you should increase your whole grain intake. Go for the brown rice or quinoa if you can. Do consider adding beans and legumes into your diet as well. If you need some sugar, go for sources like maple syrup or honey. Sugarcane juice is another worthwhile alternative.

Eliminate Processed Foods by Replacing Them with Whole and Natural Ingredients.

One of the reasons why it can be difficult to resist processed foods is because it is cheap to buy and easy to prepare. Fast food places are some of the worst sources for meals. The reason their offerings are called fast food is that people get these quick and eat them quickly.

Other types of processed foods are those that you can find in bags, boxes, or packages in the market -- cereals, chips, frozen pizza, and the like. Even some packaged frozen vegetables contain a preservative that you should avoid.

To eat clean, you should focus on finding fresh ingredients. Some of these may cost more and require more time to prep, but your body will thank you for it. Later, you'll save even more on medical bills and other expenses

Every Meal Should Consist of Carbs, Fat and Protein.

Just like in the food pyramid, having a balanced meal complete with carbs, fat, and protein is essential to a healthy well-being. Most people fail to include protein sources in their breakfast and lunch, and this practice should stop. Proteins help build muscle mass while reducing cravings making it the most important component of all.

Sugar, Salt, and Fat Should Be Controlled.

Although these are important to include in one's diet, going overboard with them will lead to excess calories and unwanted water retention. When eating clean, use these items sparingly. A proper daily diet consists of 5 to 6 small meals, not the big 3. It is quite common for people to eat breakfast, lunch, and dinner. What they fail to realize is that these big meals are not enough to fuel you throughout the day. You get so full at one point then hungry later on.

By constructing your meal plan in such a way that you get an adequate amount of calories divided into 5 or 6 smaller meals, you get a continuous supply of energy to fuel you throughout the day. You'll reduce the possibility of overheating or skip meals as a result.

Calories are Meant to be Eaten.

Juicing is all the rage these days. There are also those who opt for coffee drinks and sodas. What people fail to see is that these can add a whopping four to 500 calories to your daily diet. If you need to drink something, go for water, unsweetened tea, or skim milk. Save the calories for one of your small meals within the day.

Exercise is the Icing on the Cake.

No diet is adequate without ample activity. Even an hour of walking every day is better than having no exercise. Daily activity helps you burn calories, reduce fat, build muscle, and maintain your energy stores. It also ensures that your body continues to function like a well-oiled machine.

Dos and Don'ts of Clean Eating

Do these:

- Don't skip meals and start with breakfast one hour after waking up. Eating breakfast will provide you with the necessary nourishment and energy to kick start your day.

- Eat 5 to 6 small meals throughout the day. It means having a satisfying meal every 2 to 3 hours. By increasing your meal frequency, you will be able to battle cravings and hunger pangs much more quickly. Eating more times in a day will also help stimulate your metabolism, and this is good for weight loss.

- Every meal should have complex carbs and lean protein. It is the solution to feeling fuller longer. By concentrating on complex carbs, your body will also reduce a number of carbs converted into stored fat as these require more energy for your body to break down.

- Be careful when it comes to your portioning. You don't need any fancy equipment to control portion sizes. You can use your hands. For example, a good amount of lean protein is about the scale of a cut of meat that will fit in the palm of your hand. As for carbs or starches, consider the size of one cupped hand. For fruits and veggies, the measure of 2 cupped hands will suffice.

- Drink a lot of water. 2 to 3 liters per day is a good amount. Eating clean mixed with proper hydration is your key to balanced living.

- Eat fats, but of the healthy kind. Focus on omega-3 fats as these help brain function. You can find healthy fats in salmon and other oily fish, avocados, nuts, and even seeds. Other healthy oil options include peanut oil, olive oil, and sunflower oil.

- Increase your fiber intake. It will aid you in digestion and help you rid your body of toxins day in and day out. Fruits and vegetables are excellent sources to consider. Aside from fiber, you'll get a substantial amount of enzymes, vitamins, and nutrients from these food items too

- Pack clean food items to go. The best way to stick with a clean eating regimen is to prep and cook the food at home and then bring it with you to work. You need nothing else but a simple cooler to do this.

Avoid these:

- Processed and refined food items with preservatives and other chemicals.

- Sources of saturated and Trans fats.

- Supersized meals.

- Anti-food products (these are food items that are dense in calories but carry no significant nutritional value)

- Alcohol in excess

- Sugar-laden beverages

- Artificial food and sugars

- White flour and other over-processed food items

Not only do these things make you more at-risk for health problems but they can quickly pack on the pounds without you noticing. They make you sluggish throughout the day and prevent your body from taking in the nourishment that it requires functioning properly.

CHAPTER 2: WHAT ARE THE BENEFITS OF CLEAN EATING?

One of the main reasons why people try new diets out is because they want to lose a certain amount of weight within a period of time of time. When it comes to clean eating, it involves more of a lifestyle shift than just a short- term diet plan.

With clean eating focused on the ingestion of whole, unprocessed and fresh food items, there are significant benefits that people can achieve within a short amount of time and here are some of them.

Weight Loss

Through the years, weight gain has been a consistent problem for people of all ages. With excess weight comes a slew of health problems from diabetes to heart disease. What most people fail to realize is that their weight issues stem from their eating habits.

As the years progressed, innovations have made it more difficult for people to eat fresh foods because ready-to-eat, pre-packaged, or fast options are available on supermarket shelves and fast food outlets. Individuals who are on-the-go rarely have time to sit down for a decent meal and so they resort to these good quick fixes.

Quick, yes. Delicious, most of the time. Healthy, definitely not. These foodstuffs are laden with bad fats, bad carbs, sugars, and artificial flavorings and chemicals. It is why they taste good and can be eaten from the bag, or box.

Aside from slowing down the body, because of the excess fat and sugar, these also contribute to increased fat stores in the body due to lowered metabolism levels. They contribute to hunger pangs and cravings that result in overeating and added weight.

Clean eating keeps you full longer, and your body benefits from the influx of healthy and fresh food items that aid in proper metabolism. Paired with an adequate amount of exercise, you can lose weight without much effort.

Improved Mood

Fresh food items don't only help you shed weight but improve your mood as well. It is because your body can get sufficient nutrition, proper vitamins, and minerals when you eat clean. Based on some studies, the body produces more energy and releases more happy chemicals when you eat fruits and vegetables. The best part is that the effects of good food do not only last for a day but lingers on for about 2 to 3 days after.

Boosted Brain Function

Aside from improving your mood, the effects of fresh food items on your body also contribute to the increase in your brain function. Whereas processed food items cause you to become sluggish, clean food items help you become more focused and productive throughout the day.

Better Sleep

There is a saying that you shouldn't sleep right after eating as it will lead to indigestion and poor-quality sleep. In truth, it is the type of food items that you eat that contributes to this ill feeling. When a balanced meal is ingested for dinner, it can promote sounder sleep later on at night. Based on studies, you can even have a fruit or two before bedtime and improve your quality of sleep.

Beautiful Skin

As you eat better quality foodstuff and start exercising, your body will do away with stored toxins. After some time, you'll notice that your skin will start glowing. The saying that you are what you eat applies here.

Reduced Risk for Disease

You might feel healthy now, but your body can change without warning. It is important that you exert a certain degree of effort into assessing your daily habits, ensuring that you maintain good health until later. Get smart with the food items that you purchase, read labels, and do away with unnecessary calories. By eating clean, you'll be one step closer to longevity.

Better Exercise Experience

With increased activity, better food intake, and a lighter body, you'll start noticing the changes, like improved endurance for example, even in the way you work out. You won't get tired that easily and you're always going to be raring to go for a jog, run, or whatever it is that you love to do to sweat

CHAPTER 3: TOP 7 MYTHS OF CLEAN EATING

It's funny how some people go overboard when it comes to the diet programs they follow. It leads to the creation of myths that, instead of helping people, derail them in succeeding. These tales make the eating plan more restrictive or difficult to integrate into one's daily habit.

Unfortunately, clean eating has not been spared from these myths and here are some of the top myths you should be mindful of:

There is no such thing as "too many calories" when you are a clean eater.

When you eat clean, it just means that you are ingesting food items that have a better nutritional value compared to processed food. But this is not to say that the calorie count should be ignored. Although fresh food items are more willing and able to curb cravings and hunger pangs, if you eat too much of something, you can still gain a significant amount of weight - especially if exercise is not a part of your daily regimen.

Adopting the Clean Eating Lifestyle Means Saying Goodbye to Dairy and Gluten.

Some people are lactose intolerant while others have true allergies to gluten. In this case, countless recipes are available online. There are also tons of products available in grocery store aisles. But when you eat clean, this does not mean that removing gluten and dairy from your diet becomes a requirement. Food items that don't have either of these components are not necessarily better for you. Unless you have celiac disease or other sensitivities to these things, there is no reason to avoid them as they can be good for the body.

You can consume as much honey, molasses, and maple syrup as you want since these aren't sugar.

You will find products labeled as having no sugar even if they contain these natural sweeteners. Most people fail to realize that these are alternatives to processed sugar substances but are also sugar compounds as well.

May it be maple syrup, honey, or molasses; they react in the same way as sugar does when they are ingested. These have fructose and glucose components that give you energy but can be transformed into fat stores when consumed in large amounts, yet are not burned off by your system.

There's No Room for Bad Food If You Start Eating Clean.

Although the clean eating habit encourages people to replace processed food items with whole, unrefined ones, this does not mean that you can't indulge yourself in a cookie or two now and then. Especially for someone who has been used to eating these so-called dangerous foodstuff, eliminating them from one's diet may not be the sustainable option.

A good compromise would be to set aside around 10 to 15 percent of your diet to accommodate cheat day foodstuff. It will motivate you to stay on track and prevent you from spiraling into a junk food binge.

Go for Organic Because Everything Else Is GMO
(Genetically-Modified Organism).

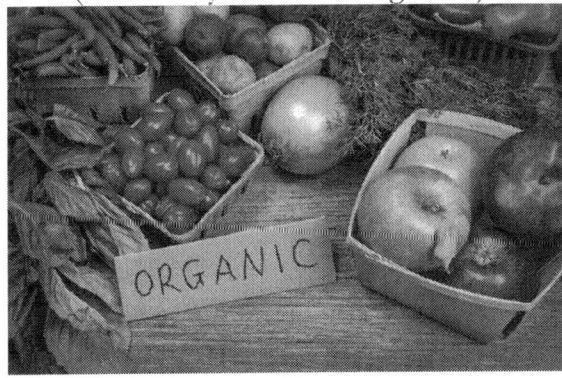

GMOs are formed in the lab with the DNA of one plant or animal being implanted into an entirely different plant or animal. Although it is evident that GMOs are not safe for you, this does not mean that all food items that are not marked as organic are automatically GMOs.

Cut Down on Sugars by Cutting Down on Fruits.

Fruits are sugary food items. It's sugar component is called fructose. In large quantities, it is undeniable that sugar is bad. But the amount of natural sugar that you can get from fruits is well within the healthy range. Aside from fructose, fruits also provide you with a sufficient amount of fiber that your body needs to maintain a healthy gut.

Aside from aiding in digestion, fiber also helps your body slow down its absorption of sugar via the bloodstream. It also gives you a fuller feeling for a longer period, reducing hunger pangs. The important thing though is that you eat fruit, not drink it as juice, or else you'll be getting way more sugar than your body needs. Keep in mind that it takes more than one piece of fruit to give you a full glass of juice.

The Terms "Clean" and "Healthy" are the Same.

Most people make the mistake of if healthy food is decent food. Sadly, this is not the case. In the same way, individual fresh snacks may not pass as healthy everyday meals. When eating clean, only focus on ingesting food items that have been proven to be good for the body; like fruits and vegetables, nuts and seeds, whole grains, and so on. If you see packaged "clean snacks" on store shelves, consider these as processed food that you can consume, but in limited quantities.

CHAPTER 4: MAKE CLEAN EATING WORK FOR YOU

Anyone can adopt the clean eating lifestyle and adjust their systems to accommodate better food items over time. In this case, it is crucial for someone like yourself to be committed to whatever it is that you are doing. It will provide you with the motivation that you need to stay on track and succeed - may it be for weight loss or other health purposes. You can make clean eating work for you. Here are some of the things that you should do, and some of the things that you should avoid, to beat the bloat, shed the weight, and become that much closer to a leaner and healthier you.

Avoiding Common Mistakes

When it comes to any new change in lifestyle, it is important that you allow for mistakes to happen. Just pick yourself up, dust yourself off, and then try again. It would also help if you had a list of common error, which those who are new to clean eating usually commit.

By knowing where others have struggled, it might be easier for you to bypass these errors

Not Pacing Yourself When You Eat

It takes about 20 minutes for your brain to realize that your stomach is filling up with food. If you eat too fast, you can consume a significant amount of calories without realizing it as you continue to feel unsatisfied despite the tremendous amount of food that you've already eaten.

By simply chewing more and slowing down the pace of every spoonful that enters your mouth, you can save tons of calories on excess food that you didn't need in the first place while putting less strain on your digestion system.

Making the Diet Excessively Strict

If you place too many restrictions on your diet, it will be unsustainable. Many people fail because they obsess over every detail. If you are intent on shifting you eating habits, you must allow yourself to adjust when you integrate new practices.

It will also be helpful if you allow even a small percentage of your food intake to accommodate things that you enjoy eating. Doing so, you will be motivated to stick with clean eating for a longer period.

Inconsistency

With anything you engage in, consistency is important to achieve desired results. Although it has been suggested that you slowly integrate clean eating practices into your lifestyle, it is important that as you progress, you focus on eating more good food.

Try to eventually break the habit of eating a healthy breakfast for example but following it with fast food meals throughout the day.

Packing on the Grains

Your body needs foods as a source of carbohydrates, fiber, or even protein but too much of anything is never a good idea. Especially when it comes to unprocessed foods, even if these are better than their refined counterparts, eating too much can lead to weight gain.

Carbo Loading Late in the Day

It is common for new dieters to stick to their plans early in the day then binge late at night. The same thing happens when you start a clean eating lifestyle.

As the willpower dwindles throughout the day, you can become susceptible to eating a lot of bad carbs, simple carbs that the body turns into fat stores, especially those made with white flour and sugar.

Not reading labels

Although the law dictates that nutritional information is printed on all packaged food items, these remain as one of the most ignored things in the world. In the world of clean eating, there is no room for mindless assumptions. It is important that you know what the food you're about to eat is made of.

It is a huge mistake not to read food labels. Even products marked as healthy, low-fat, low-sodium or what not have some form of a chemical component that might not be in line with the concept of clean eating. Also, the label contains the calorie count of the food item, and this is important information that you should know if you are counting your calories. Don't let something that is right in front of you be your downfall!

Focusing on one type of clean food at a time

When you start eating clean, do your best to adopt the entire practice, not just bits and pieces of it. Instead of focusing on taking in a whole grains, fruits, and vegetables, why not invest some time and effort ensuring that you are eating healthy balanced meals? Like what was previously mentioned, every meal needs protein, fat, carbs, fibers, fruits, and veggies.

Not Addressing Cravings and Hunger Pangs Correctly

When you adopt a clean eating lifestyle, you will start eating smaller meals more frequently during your day. It helps combat hunger pangs brought about by other diet regimens. But even as you do this, there are times when your body will want more food, and addressing these cravings can lead to some serious weight gain.

Most of the time, people who feel that they are hungry even after eating a full meal are experiencing dehydration. If the hunger pangs come, drink a glass of water. If this does not solve it, have a piece of fruit. Don't go dashing through the kitchen for that bag of cookies.

Learning to Count Calories

Aside from watching what you eat, you should also start measuring portions and calories. Calorie counting is an effective way of keeping your clean eating habits on track. Remain in mind that even if you are eating better quality food items, you still have to limit the amount of food that you ingest. In this case, overeating can still lead to significant weight gain.

Counting calories is quite simple. These days, there are plenty of apps that you can use to track how many calories you are consuming and burning in a day. If you want to go old school, just have a pen and paper with you at all times so that you can jot down all of your meals for the day, even if it is just a couple of almonds.

Proper recordkeeping is essential in this case. If you have the app, then it will automatically convert your food inputs into estimated caloric measures. If you are using a pen and paper, you can do the work manually by finding a conversion chart on the Internet. As much as possible, make it easy on your part to track calories and go for the digital option. Install the app on your phone or download a program onto your computer.

There are guides as to how many calories you need in a day given your height, weight, gender, and level of daily activity. You will also find resources online that will tell you how many calories you need to eat or burn to reach a targeted weight level.

Some people decide against counting calories mainly because it can be quite a chore, so for you to surpass this hurdle, make use of the modern innovations that you can access to make counting calories nothing but a piece of cake.

Tips to Get You Started

With clean eating, the objective is simple, and that is for you to start eating better food items and do away with options that are bad for the body. As you clean up your diet, shift your focus to consume a whole food, fresh produce rather than their processed counterparts. Different benefits come with clean eating, and it is relatively easy to get started with this change of lifestyle.

Identify a Reason as to Why You Want to Start Eating Clean.

Most people have reasons behind why they want to do certain things and know why you want to start eating better can serve as an excellent motivator for those days when you want to quit.

When you try something new, you need to put more effort into it to succeed. If you have a source of inspiration, then everything will be easier to accomplish. In this case, it is important that your primary reason for why you want to eat clean is so that you'll be healthier. Focus more on why the change will benefit you, and you'll have a better chance at succeeding.

Identify How Much You Are Willing to Commit to Succeed at It.

After you identify your reasons behind wanting to eat clean, identify a level of commitment that you can stick with. Keep in mind that you are dealing with something that involves a complete overhaul of your eating habits. Can you deal with home-prepping at least one meal a day for a week to start? Can you incorporate at least 30 minutes of exercise during your day? Don't overwhelm yourself early on. It is pretty much like goal setting wherein you need to identify reasonable levels of commitment that you can abide by as you start your journey to eating better. For some that will be 100% on the go, for others it will take longer.

Assess Your Current Eating Habits, Daily Consumption Included.

If you have your current diet laid out, then you'll know which components need changing. Do this for a week or two. Jot down your daily food consumption may it be an apple or a bag of cookies. Include information on what times of the day you are eating. Write everything down so that you can assess the gravity of your eating situation better.It will help you pinpoint the things you need to cut back on or eat more of.

You can install food journal apps on your phone or use a simple pen and paper combo, whichever is more convenient for you. After the initial recording, do your assessment and create three lists: 1) food of eating less of,
2) food to add to your diet, and 3) food to consider eliminating. Depending on how big or small these lists are will mentally prepare you for the task ahead, showing you just how much of a lifestyle change is needed.

Set Your Goals and Identify Specific Targets.

Set goals that are reasonable, those that you can achieve over time. You can create lists of short or long-term goals but start with short-termed ones at this point. Better yet have several short-term goals that will culminate into one long-term, this way before you know it you will have reached a milestone, making it seem less daunting and keeping motivation high. Using the lists you've prepared, work with various ingredients and add or remove them from your daily consumption. In this case, a slow progression is more ideal as it will not overwhelm you.

Start Shopping Smarter.

When you visit the market, be a smart shopper. It means reading labels and not hurrying when finding ingredients. Assessing the items you put in your cart will help you become a better eater. If possible, forge a new route, literally, one that will lead you to the produce section rather than the snack aisle. This way you don't have to put yourself in temptations way

Read labels and if there are plenty of things you cannot pronounce or spell, then get rid of that thing. When it comes to organic finds, do not be daunted by tag prices. Yes, better ingredients are more expensive, but these will save you tons in medical bills over time. Take your time when deciding what foods to get, shopping for these ingredients is one of, if not the most important parts of clean eating. Without the right tools, no handyman can get a job done, and it is the same with you and your diet.

Embrace The Meal-Prepping Lifestyle and Concentrate On Healthy Eating.

When you attempt eating clean, make time to prep your daily meals at home. If you set aside a couple of hours each day, you can have a cooler full of meals for the following day. Even if you work in an office, you'll always have a home-cooked meal to enjoy, a meal made with ingredients that you are acutely aware of.

At first, this will surely take some time, but after you learn the ropes, you can even try to meal prep for weeks at a time. Imagine being able to prepare a week's worth of food in a matter of hours. For recipes, a ton of them can be found online, and some sites will even draft a recipe list for you. There are in-phone apps that you can also use that'll give you prepping times, and calorie counts as well.

But it is understandable that there will be times when you need to socialize and head out for meals. If you can bring a home-prepped meal with you, then don't hesitate to do so. But if you can't, then only watch what you order. Most restaurants are very accommodating these days. You can ask the staff to do away with certain ingredients, or you can simply have them placed on the side.

Long and Short-Term Goal Setting Made Easy

With any other endeavor, it is important to set goals. Without goals, you won't have a clear direction to follow. When it comes to clean eating, it is necessary for you to have both short-term and long-term goals, all of which should not only be specific and measurable but realistic as well.

The problem why most people fail with diets or lifestyle changes is because they want unreasonably quick results without having to put in a lot of the required effort. Even with something as accommodating as a clean eating diet plan, if you don't try to shop properly or prep food at home, you won't be any closer to a healthier you.

As previously mentioned, you need not engage in significant changes right away. You can integrate better meals into your existing diet and work from there. So for your short-term goals, it can be something as simple as reducing your fast food intake from once every day to say a couple of times a week. Gradually reduce this number as you move along.

You can also replace your one-cookie-a-meal thing into one cookie per day as a midday snack. There are small things that you can start with to make it easier for your body to adapt to eating better longer. And as you progress with the integration, you can then focus on long-term goals like adopting a regular daily exercise regimen or losing a certain amount of weight by a certain date.

Set goals that you can reach and motivate yourself to take action. No pain, no gain is not the mindset that you need to have. Only consider that you need an adequate investment regarding the effort to reap the rewards.

CHAPTER 5: CHOOSING HEALTHY FOOD PRODUCTS

It is critical that you choose healthy and clean food options daily. To do this, you should at least have an understanding as to what good food is.

Good Carbohydrates versus Bad Carbohydrates

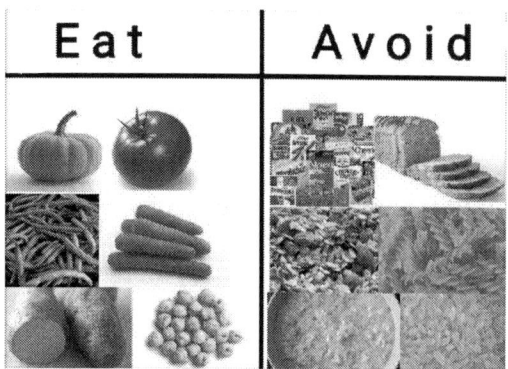

Carbohydrates are very important as they are excellent sources of energy. It does not mean though that you should carbo load every chance you get as this will lead you to gain a lot of weight.

Just like other food components, there are good carbs and bad carbs. Understanding which is which will help you make better food choices as you continue the path to clean eating. The bad carbs are the simple carbs – carbohydrate sources that are easily absorbed by your body the minute you ingest food. Good carbs are complex carbs – carbohydrates that take your body a longer time to process, giving you a more constant source of energy throughout the day.

Bad carbs are bad because they don't give your body the chance to break them down. Instead, they are immediately processed and stored as fat. They don't fill you up longer, so you end up eating more to satisfy your energy requirements. These are the carbs you find in white bread, pasta, and junk food.

As for complex carbohydrates, you can get these from whole grains and legumes. They fill you up, so you feel fuller for a longer period. These also give you excellent sources of fiber to boot. They do contain some sugar content but not a lot of it. The best part is that your body needs to work to process them correctly. In doing so, they also help raise your metabolism, helping you shed pounds as time passes.

Healthy Fats versus Bad Fats

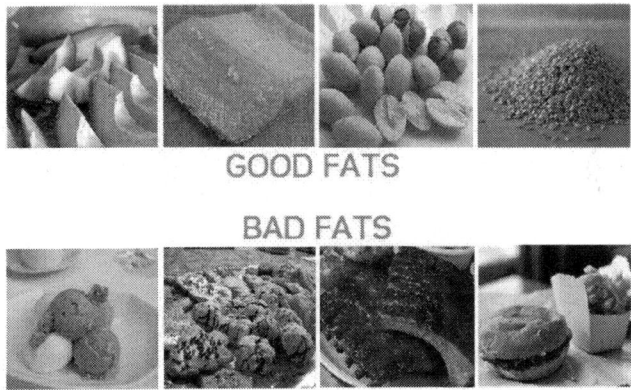

Most people do not understand the concept of fat, and this is usually because the word is associated with things like cholesterol, heart disease, stroke, obesity, and even cancer. But truth be told, there are certain kinds of fats that help the body function properly.

And with any diet, it is important that there be an adequate amount of fats, healthy fats that enter the system. There are those which you should avoid or eat in moderation and then there are the kinds that you need to achieve good health.

There are two kinds of bad fats, and these are trans and saturated fats. The primary organ these things attack is the heart, clogging it as you consume more and more of these substances over time.

Saturated fats are animal-based. Aside from dairy products, you can also find them in high-fat cuts of meat. Tran's fats, on the other hand, are Trans fatty acids that originate from partially-hydrogenated vegetable oils. Tran's fats are commonly found in processed food products like margarine, baked goods, and fast food items.

However, keep in mind that healthy fats also exist. These are healthier for the heart. Examples are polyunsaturated fat and monounsaturated fat. These kinds of fats, unlike their unhealthy counterparts, come in liquid form even when in room temperature. These include oils found in nuts, salmon, avocado, peanut butter, and olive oil, to name a few.

Healthy Proteins Versus Bad Proteins

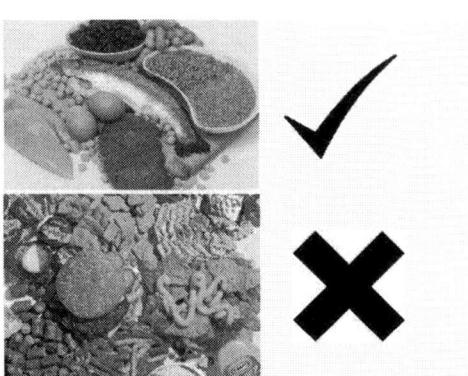

When you hear the word protein, are you one of those people who immediately think of bulging muscles and well-formed abs? Yes, protein helps develop those muscles. It also improves bodily functions, boosts strength, and gives you energy on a daily basis. It is why you should always have a right amount of protein in your diet. Eating the right amount of protein will be beneficial. Binging on it or eating too small of a sum is not advisable. Also, you should know that there are two types of protein that you should be mindful of. There is the kind of protein that is right for you, and then there are sources which you should try your best to consume sparingly or avoid altogether.

The thing about protein is that to know whether or not it is good; you should take a look at its nutrient base. Apart from this, you should also have an idea of how it was sourced – this means taking a look at how the animal was raised and farmed. Other points to consider include its omega-3 fatty acid content as well as its saturated fat component.

You should also take note of the fact that animal meat is not the only source of protein available today. There is soy which comes from plants. It is packed with nutrients and is healthy for the gut. There are also some grains, legumes, and even vegetables that give you first doses of protein. Portobello mushrooms for one are good sources of protein.

CHAPTER 6: CLEAN EATING GUIDELINES

- Avoid processed foods – they are usually high in additives and chemicals, salt and refined sugar, and that's not something you want in your system.

- Avoid refined foods – this includes refined flour, sugars, and fats. Cutting these down in your diet will produce weight loss and correct insulin levels at the same time.

- Avoid alcohol – alcohol goes into the blood which then goes into your system, disturbing the way your liver, heart, and kidneys work, so alcohol is not something you want to drink. However, if you do go out and have to drink, keep it on a shallow level.

- Avoid preservatives – read the labels of each food you buy and if it has ingredients that you can barely pronounce, don't buy it! As simple as that!

- Avoid artificial sweeteners – refined sugar is a no-no, but so are artificial sweeteners, so don't fool yourself. As their name states, they are artificial, made by humans in a lab. There's nothing natural or healthy about them.

- You and your food needs are important – choose your foods wisely and tailor your eating habits to suit your needs, according to your health, your daily tasks, or cravings. Clean eating is a highly customizable lifestyle keep that in mind all the time!

- Establish goals and eat accordingly – losing weight or gaining weight, fixing a health problem or preventing one, clean eating can make it happen!

- Veggies, veggies, veggies, that's the golden rule! Luckily, vegetables come in a wide variety, so you'll never get bored of combining them into new and appealing dishes.

- Eat fruits in moderation – unlike vegetables, fruits are sweet, and the chance of eating too much and interfering with your goal is very high. Too much sugar leads to high blood sugar levels or interferes with your hormones.

- Eat high-quality ingredients – from meat to veggies and fruits, try picking the best ingredients you can afford. It doesn't mean eating expensive foods but choosing wisely the ones that provide the most nutrients for their price.

- Eat healthy fats – fat is not the culprit for weight gain. In fact, fat is good for your brain. But always choose healthy fats – almonds, walnuts, chia seeds, avocados, eggs, extra virgin olive oil, coconut oil, good quality butter and grass-fed meat.

- Drink enough water – nothing beats pure, natural water regarding what you drink. A glass of water early in the morning is the way to go for a clean, detoxified system.

- Use less salt when cooking and read labels to find the products that have less salt.

- Cut back on caffeine – one cup of coffee a day is okay for some people, but reducing it is a good idea if you have already had certain health problems.

- Find out what works for you and stick to it, but don't be afraid to step out of your comfort zone and discover new recipes, new ingredients, new flavor combinations.

CHAPTER 7: 30-DAY CLEAN EATING MEAL PLAN

This section presents a sample meal plan that you could use for 30 days. All of the recipes in this 30-day meal plan are found in this book, and you can easily interchange methods where necessary to fit your needs and lifestyle. Additionally, there is a helpful chart which outlines the seasonality for certain fruits and vegetables. Eating can be very useful when eating clean but sticking to your family's grocery budget.

Shopping List

Fresh, Lean, Organic, And Free-Range Protein Sources

• Almond Butter

• Beef

• Chicken

• Eggs

• Fish (especially Salmon)

• Pork

• Veal

Grains, Nuts, Beans, and Seeds

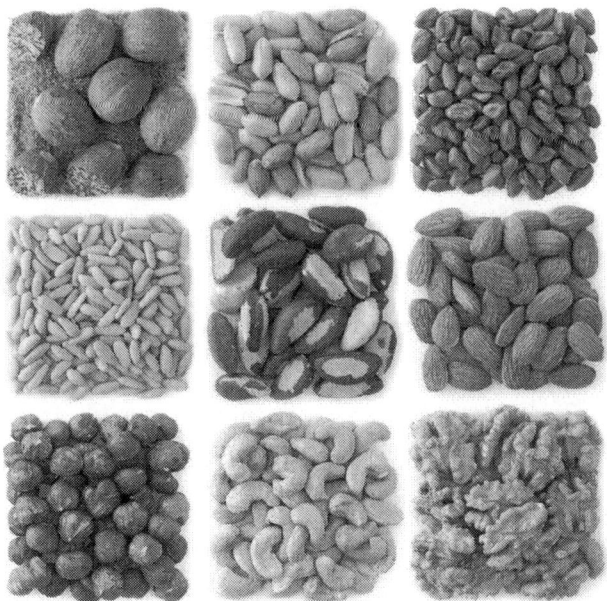

- Black beans
- Brown rice
- Cannellini beans
- Chia seeds
- Chickpeas
- Hemp seeds
- Lentils
- Millet
- Pinto beans
- Quinoa (this is also a good source of protein)
- Raw almonds
- Raw cashews
- Soba noodles (this is also a good source of protein)
- Sunflower seeds
- Tahini , Tempeh, Walnuts

Vegetables and Herbs

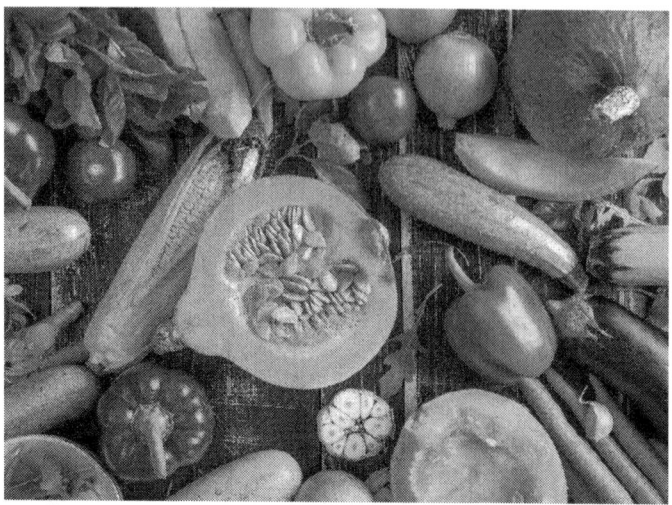

- Broccoli

- Brussels sprouts

- Cilantro

- Fennel

- Garlic

- Kale

- Lettuce

- Onion

- Other leafy greens

- Parsley

- Sweet potato

Fruits

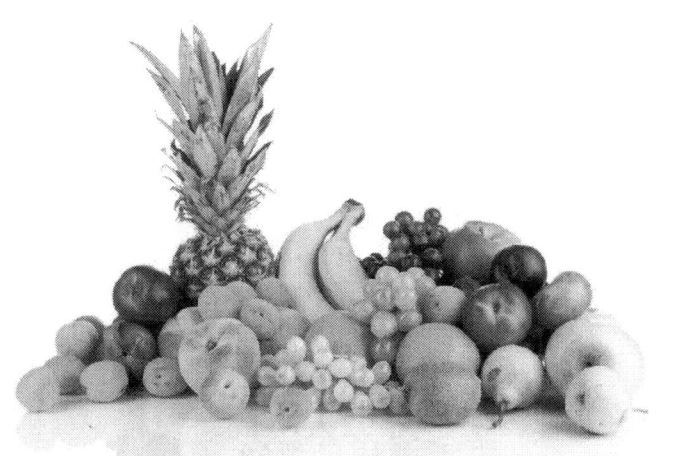

- Apples

- Avocado

- Bananas

- Berries

- Grape tomato

- Grapes

- Lemons

- Mango

- Melon

- Plum tomato

Beverages

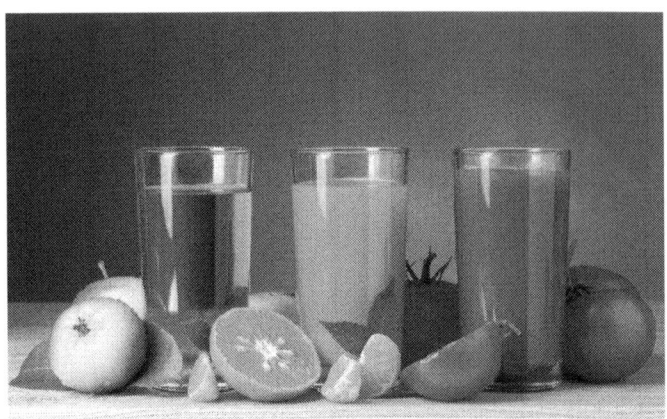

- Almond milk

- Coconut water

- Hemp milk

- Herbal teas

- Kombucha

- Water

Spices, Condiments, and Oils

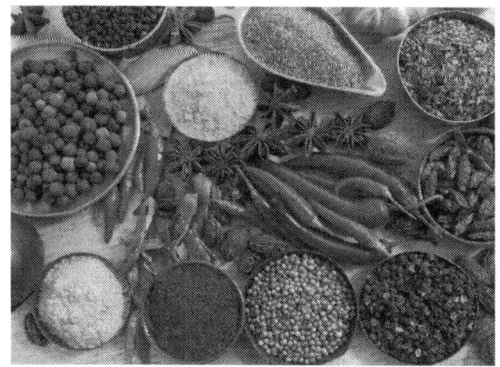

- Apple cider vinegar
- Black pepper
- Cayenne
- Cinnamon
- Coconut oil
- Dijon mustard
- Extra-virgin olive oil
- Gomasio
- Grey Celtic salt
- Hot sauce
- Maca powder
- Maple syrup
- Miso
- Pink Himalayan salt
- Red pepper flakes
- Red wine vinegar
- Sesame oil
- Stevia (you can use this as a substitute for white sugar)
- Tamari (you can use this as a replacement for soy sauce)
- Turmeric

	BREAKFAST	LUNCH	SNACK	DINNER	DESSERT
	Clean Eating 30-Day Meal Plan				
DAY 1	Brekkie Fruit Cup	Corn and Beans Pitas	Veggies with Garbanzo Dip	Glazed Potatoes and Apple	Baked Cinnamon
DAY 2	Apples and Oats	Chicken Hush Tomato Salad	Grapey Smoothie	Sauteed Zucchini	Fruitti Dip
DAY 3	Fruit Yogurt On-the-Go	Green Chili and Corn Salad	Fresh Salsa Dip	Avocado and Tortilla Chips Soup	Choco Fruit Delight
DAY 4	Boats of Papaya	Avocado Veggie Salad	Veggie Rolls	Shelled Turkey	Cold Paradise
DAY 5	Berry Banana Pancakes	Chicken Jalapeno Sandwich	Mango Pear Combo	Chix and Dumpling s	Grilled Fruit
DAY 6	Corn Tortilla Salsa	Veggie Quesadill as	Peanut Butter and Peach Pitas	Chicken Vegetable Enchiladas	Baked Peaches
DAY 7	Garlic Tomato Omelet	Turkey Greek Sandwich	Fruit and Nut Snack to Go	Veggies and Chicken Kebab	Spicy Apple Squash
DAY 8	Organic Egg Toast	Asiatic Chicken Salad	Almonds and Orange	Turkey Skillet	Apple Mini Pie
DAY 9	Sausage and Sweet Potato	Potato Herb Salad	Berry Apple Banana Drink	Lemon Chicken and Veggies	Banana Cookies
DAY 10	Cream Cheese and Lox Bagel	Apple, Raisins, and Tuna Salad	Tortilla Salsa	Veggie Combo	Almond &Chocolat e Biscotti

DAY 11	Banana Cheerios	Potato Stuffers	Egg and Apple	Sesame Chicken Recipe	Cookie Cake Bake
DAY 12	Pineapple Cottage Cheese	Mango-Avocado Chicken Salad	Pear and Cheese Snack	Chicken Stir-Fry with Sweet Mangoes	Choco Almond and Banana Morsels
DAY 13	Egg Wraps	Garbanzo Burgers	Veggie Sticks and Hummus	Turkey Meat Sauce Pasta Dish	Guiltless Cinnamon Rolls
DAY 14	Banana Waffles	Sirloin Steak Salad	Chips and Cheese Snack	Baked Potato Wedges	Golden Bananas
DAY 15	English Almond Butter Toast	Grilled Green Salad	Zucchini Salt and Vinegar Chips	Classic Fish Tacos	Choco Almond Butter Protein Chomps
DAY 16	Berries and Almonds Yogurt	Veggie Hummus Pita	Watermelon and Sunflower Snack	Turkey and Greens	Oatmeal Raisin Cookies
DAY 17	Apples and Pecans Oatmeal	Vegetable Delight	Pumpkin Sweet Quick Bread	Black Bean Chicken Burrito	Angel Cake
DAY 18	Banana Apple Oatmeal	Sausage and Ricotta Macaroni	Banana Almond Smoothie	Black Bean Dish	Banana Pumpkin Bread
DAY 19	Bacon Bread	Pizza Mexicana	Carrot Cake Muffins	Healthy Chicken Satay	Cinnamon Apple Saute
DAY 20	Blueberry Muffins	Blueberry and Salmon Salad	Tomato Cucumber Salad	Honey Lemon Chicken	Potato and Cinnamon Squares
DAY 21	Avocado Egg Prosciutto Wrap	Tuna Steak Salad	Apple Chips	Mahimahi Tortillas	Trail Mix Protein Slices

DAY 22	Cinnamon Waffles	Avocado and Turkey Wrap	Berry Frozen Dessert	Kalamata Olives Pizza	Blueberry Cake Muffins
DAY 23	Coconut Pancake	Chicken and Potato Roast	Ginger Juice Popsicles	Nutty Chicken	Choco Apple Protein Squares
DAY 24	Pumpkin and Zucchini Quick Bread	Chicken Breast with Garlic and Basil	Choco Oatmeal Bites	Roasted Salmon Fillets	Choco Avocado Pudding
DAY 25	Choco Pancakes	Turkey and Mushroo m in Sour Cream Sauce	Cocoa Fudge Pops	Turkey Shish Kebabs	Gluten-free Choco Almond Butter Bikkies
DAY 26	Coconut Lemon Pancakes	Hoisin Chicken Recipe	Strawberry Ice Lollies	Shrimp Mexicana	Oatmeal Almond Choco Cookies
DAY 27	Lavenders and Lemons Pancakes	Classic American Burger	Apple Nachos	Kale and Black Beans	Dark Choco & Black Coffee Granola Bars
DAY 28	Brekkie Bacon Veggie Pizza	Veal Zucchini Rolls	Blueberry Banana Logs	African Vegetable Dish	Cookies and Cream Chunks
DAY 29	Breakfast Coconut Power Drink	Bacon Tenderloi n Dish	Yogurt, Banana Popsicles	Spicy Bean Burgers	Healthy Apple Crisp
DAY 30	swiggy Sardines Recipe	Chops and Relish Recipe	Berry Ice Lollipops	Couscous Curry	Greek Banana

Fruit and Vegetable Guide for Every Season
If you want to stay healthy and purchase fruits and vegetables at a lower price, know what's in season through this simple guide.

Year-Round	Winter	Spring	Summer	Fall
Apples, green onion, bananas, jicama, beets, kale, bok choy, leeks, broccoli, lemons, cabbage, lettuce, limes, cactus leaves, mushrooms, onions, carrots, pineapples, parsnips, potatoes, cauliflower, celery, radishes, spinach, chili peppers, tomatillos, cucumbers, eggplant, dried fruit, canned fruits and vegetables, frozen fruits and vegetables, 100% vegetable juice, 100% fruit juice	Avocados, turnips, Brussels sprouts, tangerines, chayote squash, pears, cherimoya, oranges, grapefruit, mustard greens, guavas, kiwi fruit	Apricots, Swiss chard, artichokes, strawberries, asparagus, rhubarb, avocados, papayas, bell peppers, oranges, collard greens, mangoes, green peas, guavas, grapefruit	Apricots, papayas, pears, avocados, bell peppers, plums, cantaloupe, strawberries, cherries, corn, Swiss chard, tomatoes, grapes, Valencia oranges, grapes, yellow squash, watermelon, green beans, honeydew, green peas, zucchini, okra	Acorn squash, turnips, Brussels sprouts, tomatoes, butternut squash, tangerines, chayote squash, sweet potatoes, cherimoya, grapes, pumpkins, green beans, okra, persimmons, honeydew, pomegranates, kiwifruit

CHAPTER 8: CLEAN EATING RECIPES FOR WEIGHT LOSS

Clean Eating Breakfast Recipes

Start your day with these clean eating breakfast meals and be ready to face the day's demands with a good deal of energy!

1. Brekkie Fruit Cup

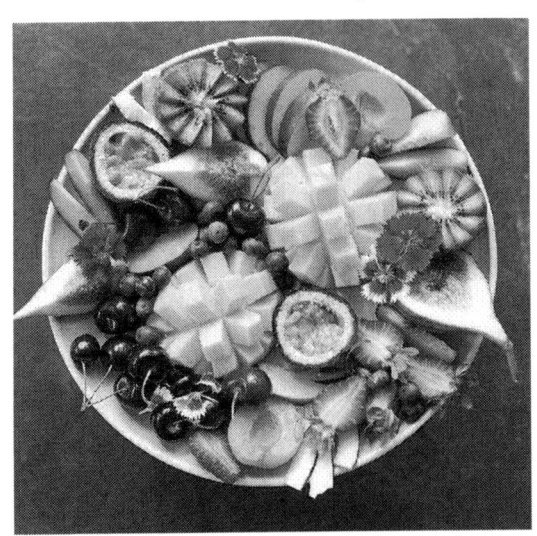

Servings: 4
Time: 5 Minutes
Ingredients:

*   One peeled and sliced banana (medium)

*   Two peeled, seeded, and sliced oranges

*   One tablespoon raisins

*   1/2 teaspoon ground cinnamon-1/3 cup low-fat vanilla

Preparation:

1. Combine all fruits in a small bowl and divide them equally into 4 cups.

2. In each bowl, add a tablespoon of low-fat yogurt.

3. Before serving, sprinkle some ground cinnamon.

2. Apples and Oats

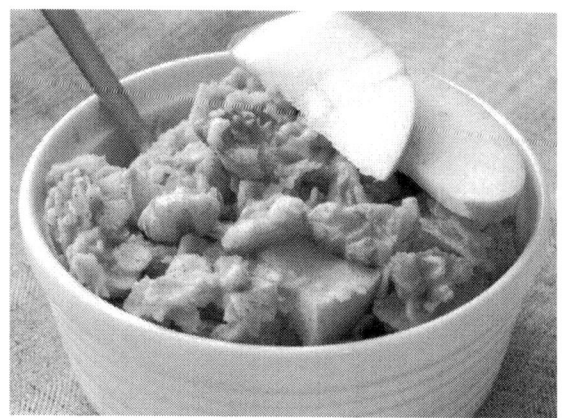

Servings: 4
Time: 2 minutes
Ingredients:

- 1 cup oats (quick-cooking)

- 1 cup 100% apple juice

- One teaspoon ground cinnamon

- One apple (large and cut into bite-sized chunks)

- 1/8 teaspoon salt (optional)

Preparation:

1. In a medium bowl, combine all ingredients.

2. Make sure the bowl is microwave-safe.

3. In the microwave, cook for 2 minutes over high setting.

4. Mix the ingredients and let cool before serving.

3. Fruit Yogurt On-the-Go

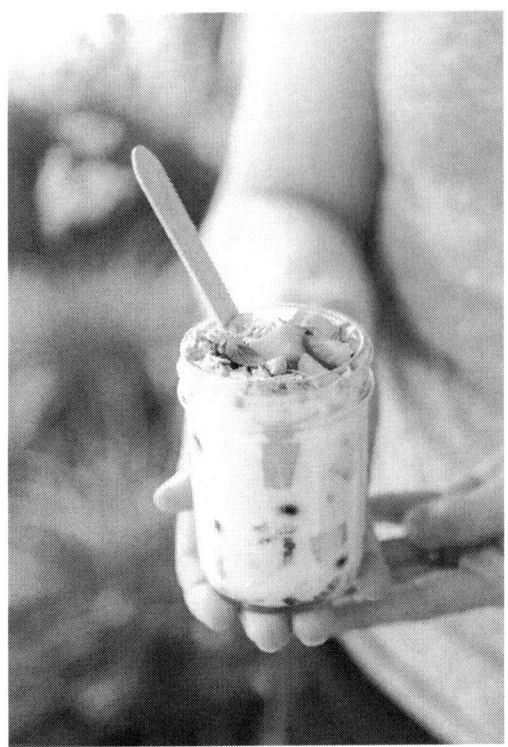

Servings: 4
Time: 5 minutes

Ingredients:

- One peeled and sliced banana (large)

- One ripe mango (peeled and cut into chunks)

- 1 cup pineapple chunks (undrained)

- 1 cup low-fat frozen yogurt (vanilla flavor)-1 cup ice cubes
  Preparation:
- In a blender container, combine all ingredients.

- Blend well until consistency is smooth.

- Then, pour mixture into cups or glasses.

4. Boats of Papaya

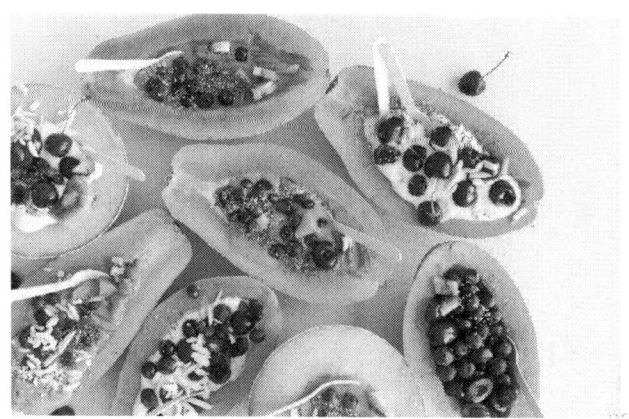

Servings: 4
Time: 10 minutes

Ingredients:

- One rinsed and peeled papayas

- One medium peeled and sliced banana

- 1 cup strawberries (sliced)

- One peeled and sliced kiwi fruit

- 1 cup low-fat vanilla yogurt

- One can drain mandarin oranges

- Two teaspoons fresh mint (chopped)

- One tablespoon honey

Preparation:

- In a medium plate, arrange papayas lengthwise.

- Put an equal amount of kiwi fruit, oranges, banana, and strawberries in each half of papaya.

- In a small bowl, mix honey, mint, and yogurt and top over fruit boats.

5. Berry Banana Pancak

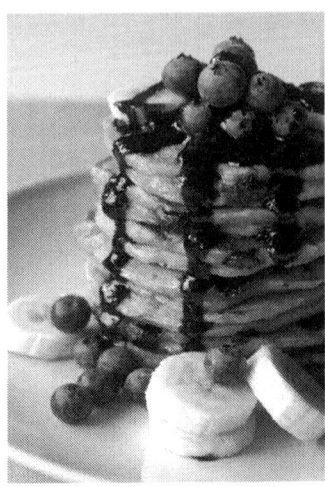

Servings: 4 servings
Time: 20 minutes

Ingredients:
- 1 cup complete pancake mix

- One large peeled and sliced banana

- nonstick cooking spray

- 1 cup water

- 1 cup unsweetened strawberries (frozen, thawed, and sliced)/Two tablespoons orange juice

Preparation:
1. In a medium bowl, mash bananas using a fork.

2. Add water and pancake mix.

3. In a skillet, pour 1 cup batter for each pancake and cook for 2 minutes for each side.

4. In another pan, cook orange juice and berries for 3 minutes.

5. Top over the pancakes.

Clean Eating Lunch Recipes
6. Corn and Bean Pitas

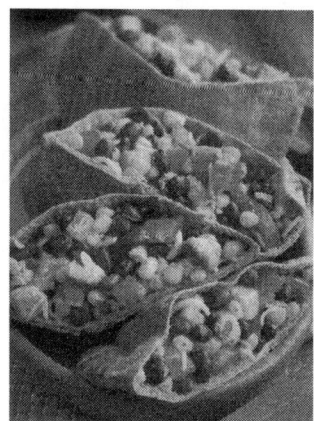

Servings: 4
Prep Time: 15

minutes

Ingredients:

- One can low-sodium black beans (15 ounces)
- 1 cup fresh, canned tomatoes
- 1 cup frozen and thawed corn
- One chopped avocado
- One teaspoon fresh parsley (chopped)
- One clove finely chopped garlic
- Two teaspoons lemon juice
- 1/4 teaspoon chili powder
- 1/8 teaspoon cayenne pepper
- 1/3 cup part-skin Mozzarella cheese (shredded)
- Two medium whole wheat pita pockets.

Preparation:

1. Rinse and drain black beans.
2. In a bowl, combine tomatoes, corn, garlic, avocado, and beans.
3. Mix and add cayenne pepper, parsley, chili powder, lemon juice, pepper, and beans.
4. Cut pita bread into two, forming four pockets.
5. Scoop your preferred amount of filling into each half of the pita bread and top with cheese.

7. Chicken Hush Tomato Salad

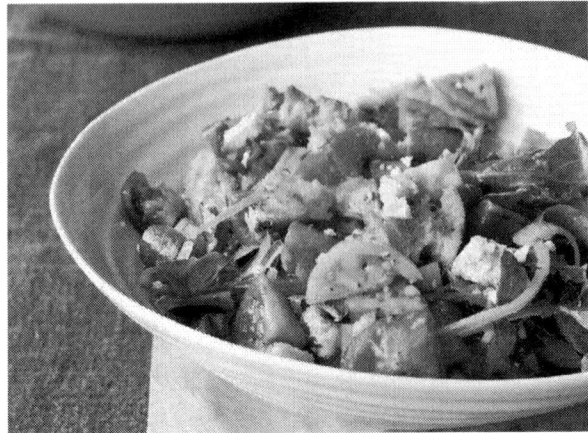

Servings: 6
Prep Time: 20 minutes
Ingredients (dressing):
- 1 cup quartered husk tomatillos
- One fresh seeded and chopped chili
- Three tablespoons dressing (light)
- 1/4 teaspoon ground black

pepper Ingredients (salad):

- 2 cups cooked and chopped chicken
- 1 cup frozen and thawed corn
- 1 cup chopped red bell pepper
- Four green sliced onions
- 1/4 cup chopped cilantro
- 1 cup chopped

carrots Preparation:

1. Pure tomatillos with ground black pepper, chili, and dressing in a
   blender.
2. Mix all ingredients for the salad and drizzle with dressing.
3. Toss well until everything is coated well.
4. Cover for 20 minutes and chill.

8. Green Chili and Corn Salad

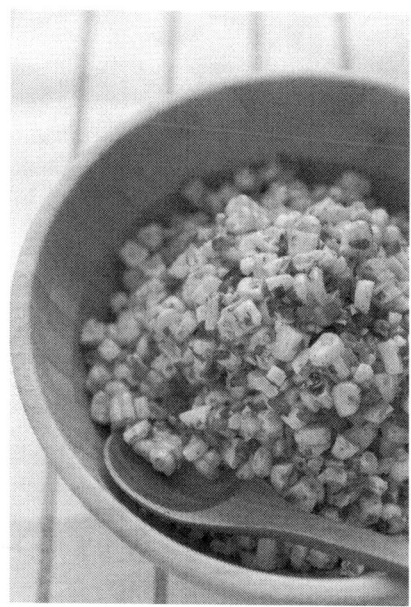

Servings: 4
Prep Time: 10 minutes
Ingredients:
* One can drain diced tomatoes with green chilies (10 ounces)

* 2 cups frozen and thawed corn

* 1/2 tablespoon vegetable oil

* 1/3 cup green onions (sliced)

* One tablespoon lime juice

* Two tablespoons fresh cilantro (chopped)

Preparation:
1. In a bowl, combine all ingredients and toss well.

9. Avocado Veggie Salad

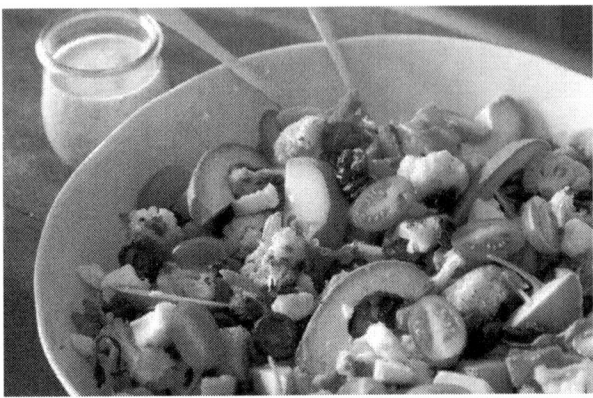

Servings: 6
Prep Time: 5 minutes
This easy to fix salad is delicious, healthy and will keep you full
all day! Ingredients:
- One large peeled avocado
- 6 cups cut mixed salad greens
- Three chopped green onions-Three medium diced tomatoes
- One small peeled and chopped cucumber
- 1/8 teaspoon salt-1/3 teaspoon garlic powder
- 1/8 teaspoon ground black pepper/Two tablespoons lemon juice

Preparation:
1. In a bowl, combine mixed salad greens, onions, tomatoes, and
   cucumber.
2. In another bowl, mix garlic powder, salt, pepper, and lemon juice.
3. Pour over salad and toss well.
4. Cut avocado in half.
5. Slice into about 1/8-inch thick wedges.
6. Assemble avocado on top of the salad and serve.

10. Chicken Jalapeno Sandwich

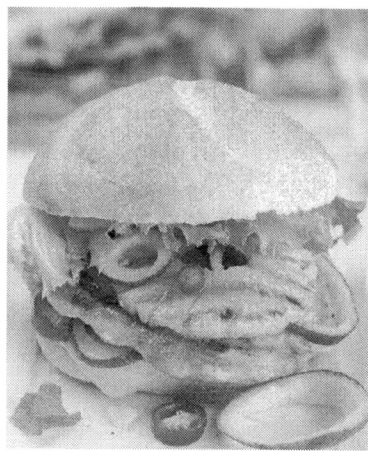

Prep Time: 15minutes

Ingredients:

- 2 cups chicken breast (cooked and shredded)
- 2 cups fresh salsa
- Four slices white onion (thinly sliced)
- One teaspoon chili powder
- 2 cups Romaine lettuce (shredded)
- jack cheese
- One fresh mashed avocado
- 2 rolls French bread (half lengthwise)/Two slices radishes

Preparation:

1. Combine chicken, 1 cup salsa, and chili powder in a bowl. Set aside.
2. Combine onion, radishes, lettuce, and cheese in another bowl. Set aside.
3. On each bread roll, spread mashed avocado and place both chicken and lettuce mixtures inside.
4. Spoon 1 cup of salsa over lettuce and close the bread.

Clean Eating Dinner Recipes

More often than not, dinner is skipped by most people, especially if they are too tired or stressed after work. They would rather rest or sleep than eat dinner. However, eating dinner is important as even when you are asleep, your body is still working. During sleep, the body starts regaining its lost energy. If you skip dinner, your body would have a hard time looking for sources of energy.

11. Glazed Potatoes and Apple

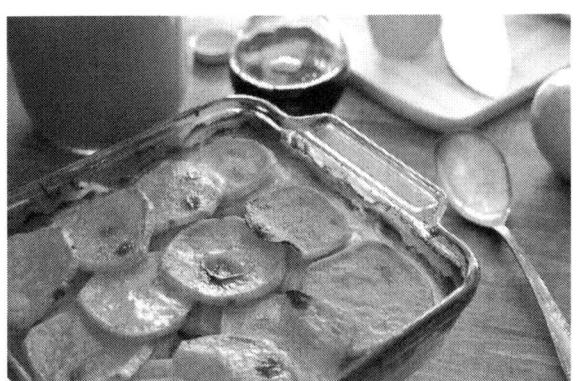

Servings: 4
Prep Time: 10
minutes Cook Time:
30 minutes

Ingredients:

- 1/2 teaspoon ground cinnamon

- 2 1/2 cups 100% apple juice (unsweetened)

- 2 pounds peeled and thinly sliced sweet potatoes

Preparation:

1. In a skillet, combine cinnamon, apple juice, and salt.

2. Add potatoes and let boil over high heat.

3. Simmer potatoes with occasional stirring for 25 minutes. Serve hot.

12. Sauteed Zucchini

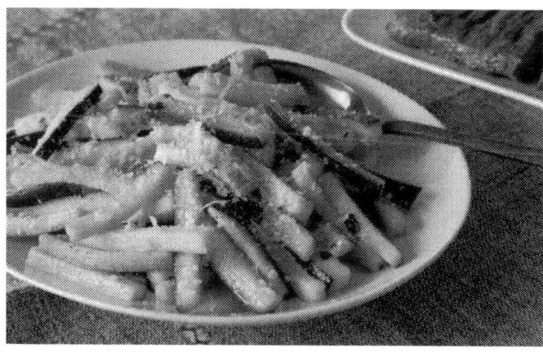

Servings: 5
Prep Time: 10
minutes Cook Time:
5 minutes

Ingredients:
- 1/2 teaspoon olive oil

- 1 1/4 pounds zucchini

- Two cloves finely chopped garlic

- One tablespoon dried oregano

- One teaspoon lemon peel (grated)

- 1/4 teaspoon ground black pepper

- One tablespoon Parmesan cheese (grated)

Preparation:
1. Cut zucchini and make four lengthwise sticks.

2. In a nonstick skillet, saute garlic and oregano over medium-high heat for 2 minutes.

3. Add lemon peel and zucchini and continue cooking for another 3 minutes. Add pepper and cheese.

13. Avocado and Tortilla Chips Soup

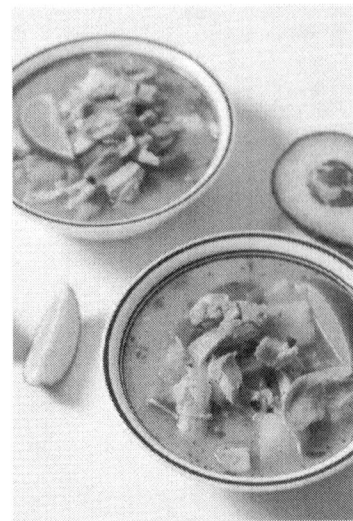

Servings: 8
Prep Time: 15
minutes Cook Time:
15 minutes

Ingredients:
- One ripe peeled, pitted and chopped avocado
- Three cans chicken broth (low-sodium)
- 1/2 bunch cilantro leaves
- Two cans condensed tomato soup (low-sodium)
- 1/2 teaspoon ground black pepper
- Three cloves finely chopped garlic
- Eight crumbled corn tortilla chips

Preparation:

1. Combine tomato soup, chicken broth, garlic, cilantro and ground black
   pepper in a pan.
2. Allow to boil and simmer for 10 minutes. Let cool and puree
   small amounts at a time in a blender.
3. Put back in the pan and add avocado.
4. Cook until avocado becomes tender.
5. Top with crumbled corn tortilla chips.

14. Shelled Turkey

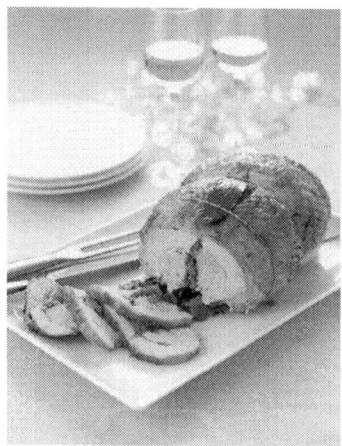

Servings: 6
Prep Time: 10
minutes Cook Time:
25 minutes

Ingredients:
- 3/4 pound ground turkey (lean)
- One medium seeded and chopped green bell pepper
- One large peeled and chopped onion
- One can diced tomatoes (without salt)
- 1/2 cup barbecue sauce (prepared)
- 1 cup canned, rinsed, and drained black beans (low-sodium)
- One teaspoon liquid smoke
- One teaspoon garlic powder
- Three bell peppers

Preparation:

1. In a skillet, brown ground turkey and drain excess fat.
2. Add onion and cook for 5 minutes.
3. Add all other ingredients except for bell peppers.
4. Simmer over medium heat for 10 minutes.
5. Cut bell peppers lengthwise. Take out the seeds. In a microwave-safe dish, put a little water and add in the bell peppers.
6. Cover and put in microwave for 5 minutes on high setting.
7. Fill bell pepper shells with turkey mixture and serve.

15. Chicken Vegetable Enchiladas

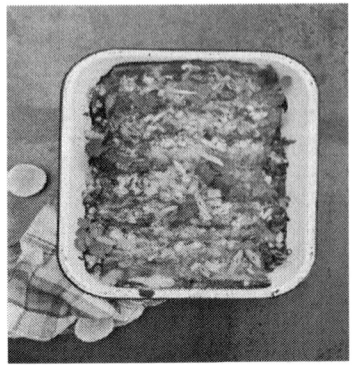

Servings: 4
Prep Time: 10
minutes Cook Time:
40 minutes

Ingredients:
- One seeded and chopped green bell pepper
- nonstick cooking spray
- One large chopped zucchini
- One large peeled and chopped onion
- 3/4 cup red enchilada sauce
- 1 cup cooked chicken breast (cut)
- Eight corn tortillas
- One cans tomato sauce (without salt)
- 2/3 cup jack cheese (reduced fats,shredded)

Preparation:
1. Set oven to 375F. Saute onion in a skillet with nonstick cooking spray.
2. Stir occasionally and cook for 5 minutes. Add zucchini and bell pepper. Cook and stir for another 5 minutes and add chicken.
3. In a small bowl, mix tomato sauce and enchilada sauce. Add half a cup to the chicken and veggie mixture.
4. Soften tortillas in the microwave and dip in the sauce.
5. Fill with chicken and vegetable mixture on one side of each tortilla.
6. Roll tortillas and arrange in a baking pan. Top with remaining sauce. Using foil, cover baking pan and put in the oven for 25 minutes.
7. When done, top with cheese and put back in the oven for 5 minutes. Serve hot.

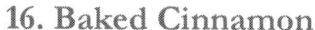

Clean Eating Desserts Recipe

After a hard day's work, you might need a nice dessert to give you some joy and let you feel relaxed. It is incredibly satisfying to give in to your sweet tooth and treat yourself. On the other hand, dessert is often a meal that is high in sugar and not appropriate for a healthy diet. In fact, desserts have a negative reputation among most health gurus. However, with a clean eating plan, you need not stay away from having a healthy dessert.

16. Baked Cinnamon

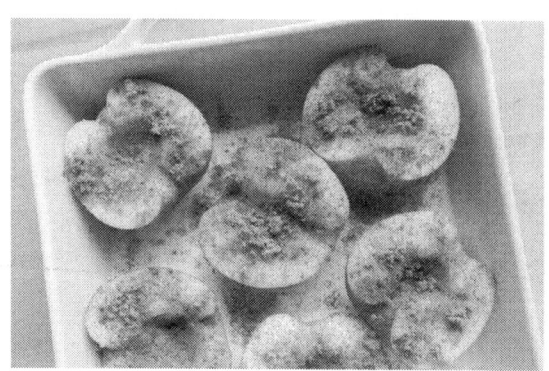

Servings: 4

Prep Time: 10 minutes / Cook Time: 10 minutes Best served with frozen yogurt and a dab of low-fat granola!

Ingredients:
- Four large cored apples
- 1/4 cup raisins -1/8 teaspoon nutmeg
- 1/2 cup 100% apple juice
- One tablespoon lemon juice
- Two tablespoons brown sugar
- 1/2 teaspoon ground cinnamon
- One teaspoon lemon peel (grated)/One tablespoon lemon juice

Preparation:
1. In a baking dish, place apples and fill with raisins.
2. In a bowl, mix all ingredients. Coat apples with the mixture and put in microwave with plastic wrap cover.
3. Remove apples from baking dish and set aside.
4. Put back baking dish in the microwave without plastic wrap cover on high setting.
5. Allow mixture to thicken for 5 minutes and drizzle over apples.

17. Fruity Dip

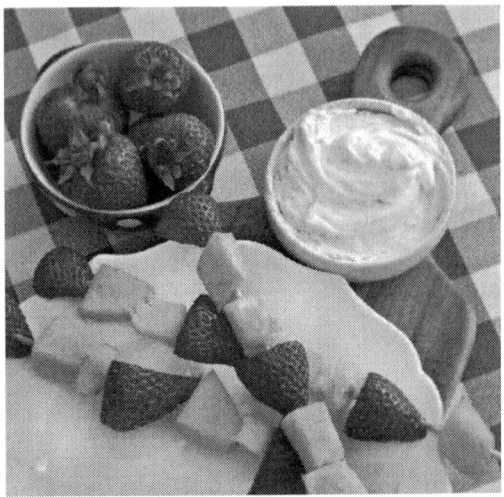

Servings: 4
Prep Time: 15 minutes

Ingredients:
- One medium cored and sliced pear

- Two medium cored and sliced red apples

- Eight large strawberries

- One medium sliced plum

- One tablespoon lime juice

- Two tablespoons 100% orange juice

- 1/2 tablespoon brown sugar/8 ounces vanilla yogurt (low-fat)
Preparation:
1. Combine lime juice, orange juice, brown sugar, and yogurt in a bowl.

2. Mix thoroughly.

3. Arrange fruits on a large plate and place the dip in the center and serve.

18. Choco Fruit Delight

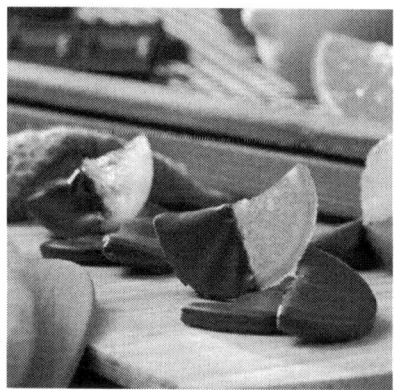

Servings: 4
Prep Time: 15
minutes Cook Time:
30 seconds

Ingredients:

* Eight large strawberries

* Two large peeled and quartered bananas or oranges

* Two tablespoons chocolate chips (semi-sweet)

* 1/4 cup chopped peanuts (unsalted)

Preparation:

1. In a safe microwave bowl, put chocolate chips and melt in the microwave on high setting.

2. Stir every 10 seconds until chocolate melts.

3. In a tray, arrange fruits and top with melted chocolate.

4. Sprinkle chopped nuts. Place the tray in the refrigerator until chocolate is hard.

19. Cold Paradise

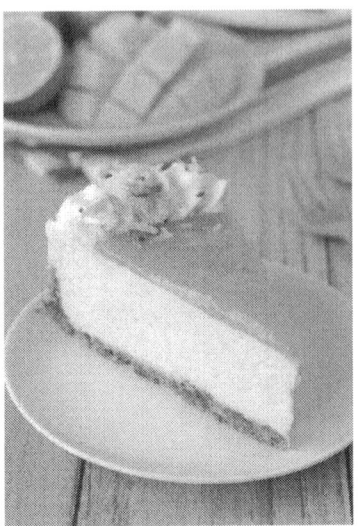

Servings: 4
Prep Time: 5 minutes

Ingredients:
- 2 cups strawberries

- One large banana

- Two ripe chopped mangoes

- 1/2 cup ice cubes

Preparation:
1. In a blender, mix all ingredients and process until texture is smooth.

2. Simply pour into four glasses. Enjoy!

20. Grilled Fruit

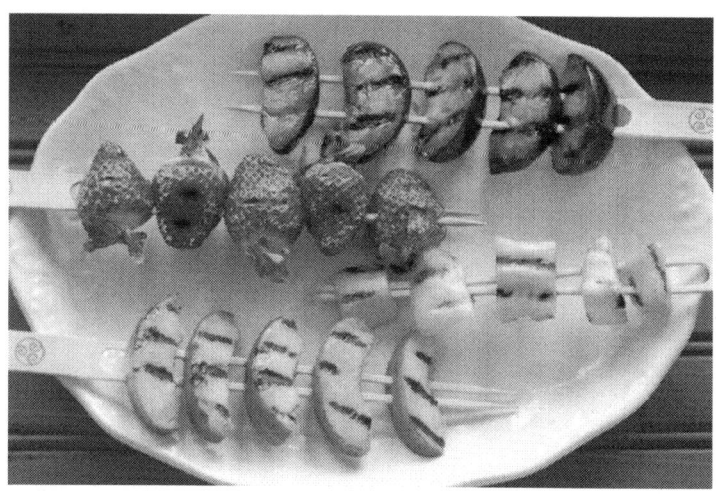

Servings: 8
Prep Time: 5
minutes Cook Time:
8 minutes
A super simple dessert to make and enjoy!

Ingredients:
• Four halved and pitted plums, peaches, or nectarines

Preparation:
1. In a covered grill, cook plums, peaches, or nectarines over indirect heat.

2. Flip after 4 minutes and continue cooking for another 4 minutes.

3. Serve and enjoy

Clean Eating Snacks Recipes

Most people avoid eating snacks because they fear these foods might contribute to weight gain or can't be part of a healthy diet. With a clean eating plan, you do not have to be afraid of eating snacks! In fact, healthy meals can even be included if you have plans of losing weight while eating clean.

The key is to opt for snacks that have a balance of protein, healthy fats, and carbohydrates. If you are concerned about calories, choose meals with approximately 100 calories or less. The goal in clean eating when it comes to snacks is to eat them halfway between meals, preferably lunch and dinner. It would keep your levels of energy stable.

Eating healthy snacks can increase mental focus and helps in sustaining your performance, be it at school or work. Most kids understand and retain lessons in school when their bodies are provided consistent with healthy food. It is best to prepare them healthy snacks that they can consume during their break time. Even adults may eat snacks in the afternoon when at work to provide them with energy; thus, they would be able to complete their tasks efficiently and quickly.

21. Veggies with Garbanzo Dip

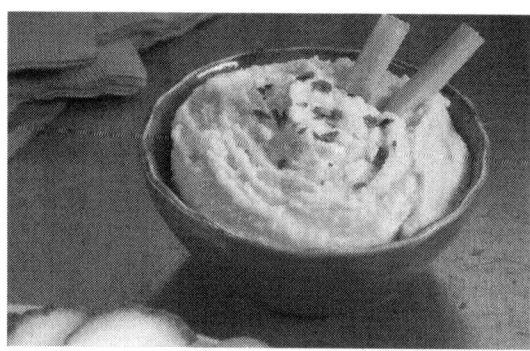

Servings: 4
Prep Time: 15
minutes
Ingredients:

- One can rinse and drained garbanzo beans or chickpeas

- 1/4 cup plain yogurt (low-fat)

- Three cloves garlic

- One teaspoon olive oil

- One tablespoon lemon juice

- 1/4 teaspoon paprika

- 1/4 teaspoon salt

- One medium sliced carrot

- 1/8 teaspoon ground black pepper

- 1/2 cup snap peasTwo medium sliced celery stalks

Preparation:

1. Combine garbanzo beans, yogurt, garlic, olive oil, lemon juice, paprika, salt, and black pepper in a food processor.

2. Pulse until texture is smooth.

3. Serve with snap peas and slices of carrot and celery stalks.

22. Grapey Smoothie

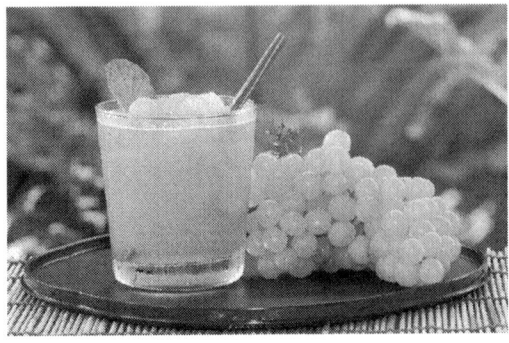

Servings: 2
Prep Time: 5 minutes
It is a hit with the kids so go ahead and let your kids enjoy this healthy smoothie!

Ingredients:
- 1 cup grapes (seedless)

- 1/2 cup frozen strawberries (unsweetened)

- 1/2 cup cherries (frozen)

- 1/2 cup slices of banana

- 1/2 cup slices of orange

Preparation:
1. In a blender, combine all ingredients and blend until smooth. Serve in glasses. (Note: It is best to freeze grapes before blending.

2. Rinse grapes and dry using a paper towel.

3. Spread on a pie pan in single layer. Cover and put in the freezer for 2 hours.)

23. Free Salsa Dip

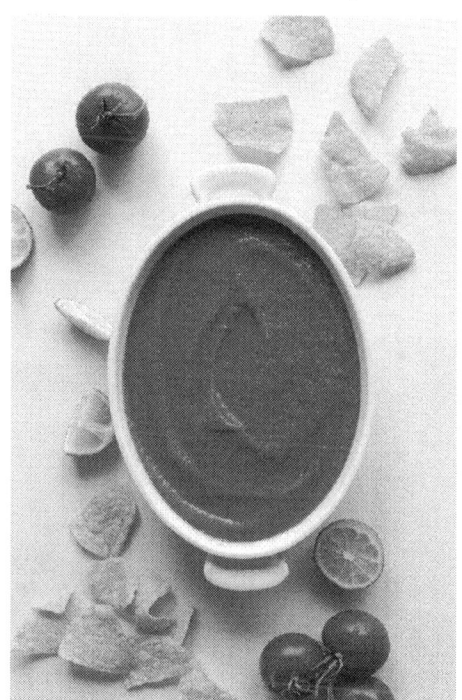

Servings: 6
Prep Time: 20 minutes
Try dipping veggies and low-sodium tortillas into this tasty salsa!

Ingredients:
- 1 pound chopped ripe tomatoes

- 1/3 cup fresh cilantro (chopped)

- 1 1/2 cups onion (chopped)

- Two tablespoons lime juice

- Three seeded and chopped jalapeno peppers

- Two cloves finely chopped garlic-1/4 teaspoon salt

Preparation:
1. Simply mix all ingredients in a bowl and serve immediately or refrigerate with cover for up to 3 days.

24. Veggie Rolls

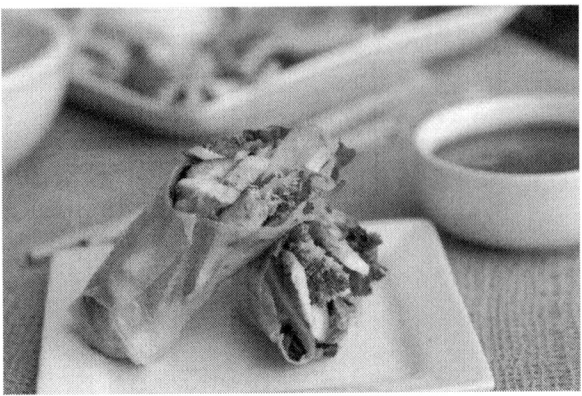

Servings: 4
Prep Time: 20 minutes

Ingredients:
- Eight tablespoons cream cheese (non-fat)

- Four tortillas (whole wheat)

- 1 cup tomato (chopped)

- 2 cups fresh spinach (chopped)

- 1/2 cup cucumber (chopped)

- 1/2 cup bell pepper (cut; any color)

- 1/4 cup drained ripe olives (sliced)

- 1/4 cup canned green chiles (diced)

Preparation:
1. In each tortilla, spread two tablespoons of cream cheese.

2. Put equal amounts of vegetables on top of cream cheese and roll tortilla up. Serve.

25. Mango Pear Combo

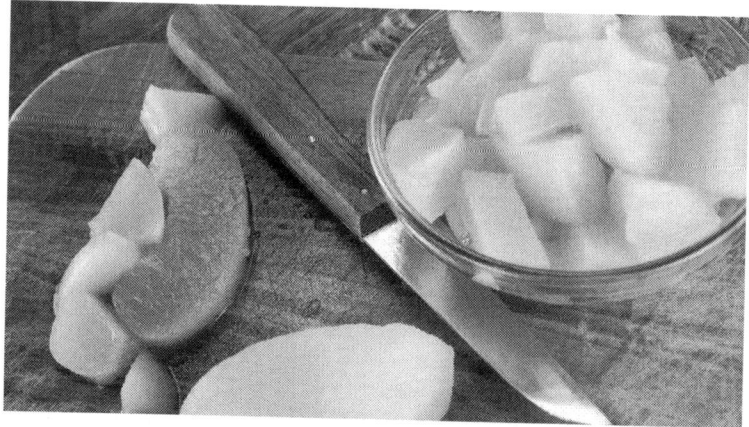

Servings: 6
Prep Time: 30
minutes

Ingredients:

- 1/2 peeled and seeded mango (chunked)

- Two medium peeled and cored pears (chunked)

- 1/3 cup red bell pepper (finely chopped)

- 1/3 cup yellow bell pepper (finely chopped)

- One small seeded and finely chopped jalapeno pepper

- 1/4 cup red onion (finely chopped)

- Two teaspoons vegetable oil

- Three tablespoon fresh cilantro (finely chopped), juice lime, sault

Preparation

1. In a bowl, mix all ingredients and put in a covered container.

2. Refrigerate for 30 minutes up to 3 hours.

3. Serve salsa with quesadillas or tortilla chips.

4. It is also best served with grilled meat or roasted fish.

CONCLUSION

What does is it mean to be on a clean eating diet? Does it mean that we are only eating organic? Vegetarian? Vegan? Raw? There are many ways of eating clean. Fast food, processed food, sugar and too much flour is not healthy for you. These have addicting substances in them. They also slow your body's metabolism down. These two reasons are causing you to gain weight. 2/3 of North Americans are now considered overweight, obese and up to morbidly obese.

By eating clean, you eliminate anything processed. What you are eating is real food. When you eat real food you don't have to count calories. Junk food is out of the question. How can you tell whether you are eating clean? There is one main way, and that is: how you feel.

A clean eating diet is a lifestyle. It is having a healthy relationship with your food. When doing a clean eating diet, it changes the way you look at the world. It can be fun and exciting. Thank you for purchasing this book I hope you will apply the acquired knowledge productively.

Made in the USA
Middletown, DE
08 August 2018